The Medical Health Checklist5

Copyright: Published in the United States by Rita L. Spears
Published March 2017

All rights reserved. No part of this publication may be reproduced, stored in retrieval system, copied in any form or by any means, electronic, mechanical, photocopying, recording or otherwise transmitted without written permission from the publisher. Please do not participate in or encourage piracy of this material in any way. You must not circulate this book in any format. Rita L. Spears does not control or direct users' actions and is not responsible for the information or content shared, harm and/or actions of the book readers.

ISBN-13: 978-1544794259

ISBN-10: 1544794258

Medical Consent Form

In case of emergency, _____ has my consent to authorize medical care for my child(ren) listed below:

_____   _____

_____   _____

_____   _____

Our family physician is: _____

His/Her address is: _____

His/Her telephone # is: _____

Our hospital preference is: _____

Allergies: _____

Contact me immediately at: _____

If unable to contact me, please call:

_____ @ _____
        Name   Telephone

_____ @ _____
        Name   Telephone

Signed by

Name: _____

Address: _____

Telephone: _____

Date: _____

Medical Consent Form

In case of emergency, _____ has my consent to authorize medical care for my child(ren) listed below:

_____   _____

_____   _____

_____   _____

Our family physician is: _____

His/Her address is: _____

His/Her telephone # is: _____

Our hospital preference is: _____

Allergies: _____

Contact me immediately at: _____

If unable to contact me, please call:

_____ @ _____
              Name   Telephone

_____ @ _____
              Name   Telephone

Signed by

Name: _____

Address: _____

Telephone: _____

Date: _____

Medical Consent Form

In case of emergency, _____ has my consent to authorize medical care for my child(ren) listed below:

_____ _____

_____ _____

_____ _____

Our family physician is: _____

His/Her address is: _____

His/Her telephone # is: _____

Our hospital preference is: _____

Allergies: _____

Contact me immediately at: _____

If unable to contact me, please call:

_____ @ _____
              Name   Telephone

_____ @ _____
              Name   Telephone

Signed by

Name: _____

Address: _____

Telephone: _____

Date: _____

Medical Consent Form

In case of emergency, _____ has my consent to authorize medical care for my child(ren) listed below:

_____   _____

_____   _____

_____   _____

Our family physician is: _____

His/Her address is: _____

His/Her telephone # is: _____

Our hospital preference is: _____

Allergies: _____

Contact me immediately at: _____

If unable to contact me, please call:

_____ @ _____
            Name   Telephone

_____ @ _____
            Name   Telephone

Signed by

Name: _____

Address: _____

Telephone: _____

Date: _____

Medical Consent Form

In case of emergency, _____ has my consent to authorize medical care for my child(ren) listed below:

_____   _____

_____   _____

_____   _____

Our family physician is: _____

His/Her address is: _____

His/Her telephone # is: _____

Our hospital preference is: _____

Allergies: _____

Contact me immediately at: _____

If unable to contact me, please call:

_____ @ _____
              Name   Telephone

_____ @ _____
              Name   Telephone

Signed by

Name: _____

Address: _____

Telephone: _____

Date: _____

Medical Consent Form

In case of emergency, _____ has my consent to authorize medical care for my child(ren) listed below:

_____   _____

_____   _____

_____   _____

Our family physician is: _____

His/Her address is: _____

His/Her telephone # is: _____

Our hospital preference is: _____

Allergies: _____

Contact me immediately at: _____

If unable to contact me, please call:

_____ @ _____
             Name   Telephone

_____ @ _____
             Name   Telephone

Signed by

Name: _____

Address: _____

Telephone: _____

Date: _____

Medical Consent Form

In case of emergency, _____ has my consent to authorize medical care for my child(ren) listed below:

_____   _____

_____   _____

_____   _____

Our family physician is: _____

His/Her address is: _____

His/Her telephone # is: _____

Our hospital preference is: _____

Allergies: _____

Contact me immediately at: _____

If unable to contact me, please call:

_____ @ _____
         Name   Telephone

_____ @ _____
         Name   Telephone

Signed by

Name: _____

Address: _____

Telephone: _____

Date: _____

Medical Consent Form

In case of emergency, _____ has my consent to authorize medical care for my child(ren) listed below:

_____   _____

_____   _____

_____   _____

Our family physician is: _____

His/Her address is: _____

His/Her telephone # is: _____

Our hospital preference is: _____

Allergies: _____

Contact me immediately at: _____

If unable to contact me, please call:

_____ @ _____
            Name   Telephone

_____ @ _____
            Name   Telephone

Signed by

Name: _____

Address: _____

Telephone: _____

Date: _____

Medical Consent Form

In case of emergency, _____ has my consent to authorize medical care for my child(ren) listed below:

_____   _____

_____   _____

_____   _____

Our family physician is: _____

His/Her address is: _____

His/Her telephone # is: _____

Our hospital preference is: _____

Allergies: _____

Contact me immediately at: _____

If unable to contact me, please call:

_____ @ _____
              Name   Telephone

_____ @ _____
              Name   Telephone

Signed by

Name: _____

Address: _____

Telephone: _____

Date: _____

Medical Consent Form

In case of emergency, _____ has my consent to authorize medical care for my child(ren) listed below:

_____   _____

_____   _____

_____   _____

Our family physician is: _____

His/Her address is: _____

His/Her telephone # is: _____

Our hospital preference is: _____

Allergies: _____

Contact me immediately at: _____

If unable to contact me, please call:

_____ @ _____
               Name   Telephone

_____ @ _____
               Name   Telephone

Signed by

Name: _____

Address: _____

Telephone: _____

Date: _____

Medical Consent Form

In case of emergency, _____ has my consent to authorize medical care for my child(ren) listed below:

_____   _____

_____   _____

_____   _____

Our family physician is: _____

His/Her address is: _____

His/Her telephone # is: _____

Our hospital preference is: _____

Allergies: _____

Contact me immediately at: _____

If unable to contact me, please call:

_____ @ _____
  Name   Telephone

_____ @ _____
  Name   Telephone

Signed by

Name: _____

Address: _____

Telephone: _____

Date: _____

Medical Consent Form

In case of emergency, _____ has my consent to authorize medical care for my child(ren) listed below:

_____   _____

_____   _____

_____   _____

Our family physician is: _____

His/Her address is: _____

His/Her telephone # is: _____

Our hospital preference is: _____

Allergies: _____

Contact me immediately at: _____

If unable to contact me, please call:

_____ @ _____
         Name   Telephone

_____ @ _____
         Name   Telephone

Signed by

Name: _____

Address: _____

Telephone: _____

Date: _____

Medical Consent Form

In case of emergency, _____ has my consent to authorize medical care for my child(ren) listed below:

_____ _____

_____ _____

_____ _____

Our family physician is: _____

His/Her address is: _____

His/Her telephone # is: _____

Our hospital preference is: _____

Allergies: _____

Contact me immediately at: _____

If unable to contact me, please call:

_____ @ _____
            Name   Telephone

_____ @ _____
            Name   Telephone

Signed by

Name: _____

Address: _____

Telephone: _____

Date: _____

Medical Consent Form

In case of emergency, _____ has my consent to authorize medical care for my child(ren) listed below:

_____   _____

_____   _____

_____   _____

Our family physician is: _____

His/Her address is: _____

His/Her telephone # is: _____

Our hospital preference is: _____

Allergies: _____

Contact me immediately at: _____

If unable to contact me, please call:

_____ @ _____
         Name   Telephone

_____ @ _____
         Name   Telephone

Signed by

Name: _____

Address: _____

Telephone: _____

Date: _____

Medical Consent Form

In case of emergency, _____ has my consent to authorize medical care for my child(ren) listed below:

_____   _____

_____   _____

_____   _____

Our family physician is: _____

His/Her address is: _____

His/Her telephone # is: _____

Our hospital preference is: _____

Allergies: _____

Contact me immediately at: _____

If unable to contact me, please call:

_____ @ _____
           Name   Telephone

_____ @ _____
           Name   Telephone

Signed by

Name: _____

Address: _____

Telephone: _____

Date: _____

Medical Consent Form

In case of emergency, _____ has my consent to authorize medical care for my child(ren) listed below:

_____   _____

_____   _____

_____   _____

Our family physician is: _____

His/Her address is: _____

His/Her telephone # is: _____

Our hospital preference is: _____

Allergies: _____

Contact me immediately at: _____

If unable to contact me, please call:

_____ @ _____
         Name   Telephone

_____ @ _____
         Name   Telephone

Signed by

Name: _____

Address: _____

Telephone: _____

Date: _____

Medical Consent Form

In case of emergency, _____ has my consent to authorize medical care for my child(ren) listed below:

_____   _____

_____   _____

_____   _____

Our family physician is: _____

His/Her address is: _____

His/Her telephone # is: _____

Our hospital preference is: _____

Allergies: _____

Contact me immediately at: _____

If unable to contact me, please call:

_____ @ _____
               Name   Telephone

_____ @ _____
               Name   Telephone

Signed by

Name: _____

Address: _____

Telephone: _____

Date: _____

Medical Consent Form

In case of emergency, _____ has my consent to authorize medical care for my child(ren) listed below:

_____   _____

_____   _____

_____   _____

Our family physician is: _____

His/Her address is: _____

His/Her telephone # is: _____

Our hospital preference is: _____

Allergies: _____

Contact me immediately at: _____

If unable to contact me, please call:

_____ @ _____
         Name   Telephone

_____ @ _____
         Name   Telephone

Signed by

Name: _____

Address: _____

Telephone: _____

Date: _____

Medical Consent Form

In case of emergency, _____ has my consent to authorize medical care for my child(ren) listed below:

_____   _____

_____   _____

_____   _____

Our family physician is: _____

His/Her address is: _____

His/Her telephone # is: _____

Our hospital preference is: _____

Allergies: _____

Contact me immediately at: _____

If unable to contact me, please call:

_____ @ _____
           Name   Telephone

_____ @ _____
           Name   Telephone

Signed by

Name: _____

Address: _____

Telephone: _____

Date: _____

Medical Consent Form

In case of emergency, _____ has my consent to authorize medical care for my child(ren) listed below:

_____   _____

_____   _____

_____   _____

Our family physician is: _____

His/Her address is: _____

His/Her telephone # is: _____

Our hospital preference is: _____

Allergies: _____

Contact me immediately at: _____

If unable to contact me, please call:

_____ @ _____
          Name   Telephone

_____ @ _____
          Name   Telephone

Signed by

Name: _____

Address: _____

Telephone: _____

Date: _____

Medical Consent Form

In case of emergency, _____ has my consent to authorize medical care for my child(ren) listed below:

_____   _____

_____   _____

_____   _____

Our family physician is: _____

His/Her address is: _____

His/Her telephone # is: _____

Our hospital preference is: _____

Allergies: _____

Contact me immediately at: _____

If unable to contact me, please call:

_____ @ _____
        Name   Telephone

_____ @ _____
        Name   Telephone

Signed by

Name: _____

Address: _____

Telephone: _____

Date: _____

Medical Consent Form

In case of emergency, _____ has my consent to authorize medical care for my child(ren) listed below:

_____   _____

_____   _____

_____   _____

Our family physician is: _____

His/Her address is: _____

His/Her telephone # is: _____

Our hospital preference is: _____

Allergies: _____

Contact me immediately at: _____

If unable to contact me, please call:

_____ @ _____
            Name   Telephone

_____ @ _____
            Name   Telephone

Signed by

Name: _____

Address: _____

Telephone: _____

Date: _____

Medical Consent Form

In case of emergency, _____ has my consent to authorize medical care for my child(ren) listed below:

_____   _____

_____   _____

_____   _____

Our family physician is: _____

His/Her address is: _____

His/Her telephone # is: _____

Our hospital preference is: _____

Allergies: _____

Contact me immediately at: _____

If unable to contact me, please call:

_____ @ _____
         Name   Telephone

_____ @ _____
         Name   Telephone

Signed by

Name: _____

Address: _____

Telephone: _____

Date: _____

Medical Consent Form

In case of emergency, _____ has my consent to authorize medical care for my child(ren) listed below:

_____   _____

_____   _____

_____   _____

Our family physician is: _____

His/Her address is: _____

His/Her telephone # is: _____

Our hospital preference is: _____

Allergies: _____

Contact me immediately at: _____

If unable to contact me, please call:

_____ @ _____
              Name   Telephone

_____ @ _____
              Name   Telephone

Signed by

Name: _____

Address: _____

Telephone: _____

Date: _____

Medical Consent Form

In case of emergency, _____ has my consent to authorize medical care for my child(ren) listed below:

_____   _____

_____   _____

_____   _____

Our family physician is: _____

His/Her address is: _____

His/Her telephone # is: _____

Our hospital preference is: _____

Allergies: _____

Contact me immediately at: _____

If unable to contact me, please call:

_____ @ _____
         Name   Telephone

_____ @ _____
         Name   Telephone

Signed by

Name: _____

Address: _____

Telephone: _____

Date: _____

Medical Consent Form

In case of emergency, _____ has my consent to authorize medical care for my child(ren) listed below:

_____   _____

_____   _____

_____   _____

Our family physician is: _____

His/Her address is: _____

His/Her telephone # is: _____

Our hospital preference is: _____

Allergies: _____

Contact me immediately at: _____

If unable to contact me, please call:

_____ @ _____
        Name   Telephone

_____ @ _____
        Name   Telephone

Signed by

Name: _____

Address: _____

Telephone: _____

Date: _____

Medical Consent Form

In case of emergency, _____ has my consent to authorize medical care for my child(ren) listed below:

_____   _____

_____   _____

_____   _____

Our family physician is: _____

His/Her address is: _____

His/Her telephone # is: _____

Our hospital preference is: _____

Allergies: _____

Contact me immediately at: _____

If unable to contact me, please call:

_____ @ _____
    Name   Telephone

_____ @ _____
    Name   Telephone

Signed by

Name: _____

Address: _____

Telephone: _____

Date: _____

Medical Consent Form

In case of emergency, _____ has my consent to authorize medical care for my child(ren) listed below:

_____   _____

_____   _____

_____   _____

Our family physician is: _____

His/Her address is: _____

His/Her telephone # is: _____

Our hospital preference is: _____

Allergies: _____

Contact me immediately at: _____

If unable to contact me, please call:

_____ @ _____
            Name   Telephone
_____ @ _____
            Name   Telephone

Signed by

Name: _____

Address: _____

Telephone: _____

Date: _____

Medical Consent Form

In case of emergency, _____ has my consent to authorize medical care for my child(ren) listed below:

_____   _____

_____   _____

_____   _____

Our family physician is: _____

His/Her address is: _____

His/Her telephone # is: _____

Our hospital preference is: _____

Allergies: _____

Contact me immediately at: _____

If unable to contact me, please call:

_____ @ _____
              Name   Telephone

_____ @ _____
              Name   Telephone

Signed by

Name: _____

Address: _____

Telephone: _____

Date: _____

Medical Consent Form

In case of emergency, _____ has my consent to authorize medical care for my child(ren) listed below:

_____   _____

_____   _____

_____   _____

Our family physician is: _____

His/Her address is: _____

His/Her telephone # is: _____

Our hospital preference is: _____

Allergies: _____

Contact me immediately at: _____

If unable to contact me, please call:

_____ @ _____
              Name   Telephone

_____ @ _____
              Name   Telephone

Signed by

Name: _____

Address: _____

Telephone: _____

Date: _____

Medical Consent Form

In case of emergency, _____ has my consent to authorize medical care for my child(ren) listed below:

_____   _____

_____   _____

_____   _____

Our family physician is: _____

His/Her address is: _____

His/Her telephone # is: _____

Our hospital preference is: _____

Allergies: _____

Contact me immediately at: _____

If unable to contact me, please call:

_____ @ _____
         Name   Telephone

_____ @ _____
         Name   Telephone

Signed by

Name: _____

Address: _____

Telephone: _____

Date: _____

Medical Consent Form

In case of emergency, _____ has my consent to authorize medical care for my child(ren) listed below:

_____   _____

_____   _____

_____   _____

Our family physician is: _____

His/Her address is: _____

His/Her telephone # is: _____

Our hospital preference is: _____

Allergies: _____

Contact me immediately at: _____

If unable to contact me, please call:

_____ @ _____
             Name   Telephone

_____ @ _____
             Name   Telephone

Signed by

Name: _____

Address: _____

Telephone: _____

Date: _____

Medical Consent Form

In case of emergency, _____ has my consent to authorize medical care for my child(ren) listed below:

_____   _____

_____   _____

_____   _____

Our family physician is: _____

His/Her address is: _____

His/Her telephone # is: _____

Our hospital preference is: _____

Allergies: _____

Contact me immediately at: _____

If unable to contact me, please call:

_____ @ _____
         Name   Telephone

_____ @ _____
         Name   Telephone

Signed by

Name: _____

Address: _____

Telephone: _____

Date: _____

Medical Consent Form

In case of emergency, _____ has my consent to authorize medical care for my child(ren) listed below:

_____   _____

_____   _____

_____   _____

Our family physician is: _____

His/Her address is: _____

His/Her telephone # is: _____

Our hospital preference is: _____

Allergies: _____

Contact me immediately at: _____

If unable to contact me, please call:

_____ @ _____
         Name   Telephone

_____ @ _____
         Name   Telephone

Signed by

Name: _____

Address: _____

Telephone: _____

Date: _____

Medical Consent Form

In case of emergency, _____ has my consent to authorize medical care for my child(ren) listed below:

_____   _____

_____   _____

_____   _____

Our family physician is: _____

His/Her address is: _____

His/Her telephone # is: _____

Our hospital preference is: _____

Allergies: _____

Contact me immediately at: _____

If unable to contact me, please call:

_____ @ _____
          Name   Telephone

_____ @ _____
          Name   Telephone

Signed by

Name: _____

Address: _____

Telephone: _____

Date: _____

Medical Consent Form

In case of emergency, _____ has my consent to authorize medical care for my child(ren) listed below:

_____   _____

_____   _____

_____   _____

Our family physician is: _____

His/Her address is: _____

His/Her telephone # is: _____

Our hospital preference is: _____

Allergies: _____

Contact me immediately at: _____

If unable to contact me, please call:

_____ @ _____
          Name   Telephone

_____ @ _____
          Name   Telephone

Signed by

Name: _____

Address: _____

Telephone: _____

Date: _____

Medical Consent Form

In case of emergency, _____ has my consent to authorize medical care for my child(ren) listed below:

_____   _____

_____   _____

_____   _____

Our family physician is: _____

His/Her address is: _____

His/Her telephone # is: _____

Our hospital preference is: _____

Allergies: _____

Contact me immediately at: _____

If unable to contact me, please call:

_____ @ _____
          Name   Telephone

_____ @ _____
          Name   Telephone

Signed by

Name: _____

Address: _____

Telephone: _____

Date: _____

Medical Consent Form

In case of emergency, _____ has my consent to authorize medical care for my child(ren) listed below:

_____   _____

_____   _____

_____   _____

Our family physician is: _____

His/Her address is: _____

His/Her telephone # is: _____

Our hospital preference is: _____

Allergies: _____

Contact me immediately at: _____

If unable to contact me, please call:

_____ @ _____
            Name   Telephone

_____ @ _____
            Name   Telephone

Signed by

Name: _____

Address: _____

Telephone: _____

Date: _____

Medical Consent Form

In case of emergency, _____ has my consent to authorize medical care for my child(ren) listed below:

_____ _____

_____ _____

_____ _____

Our family physician is: _____

His/Her address is: _____

His/Her telephone # is: _____

Our hospital preference is: _____

Allergies: _____

Contact me immediately at: _____

If unable to contact me, please call:

_____ @ _____
          Name   Telephone

_____ @ _____
          Name   Telephone

Signed by

Name: _____

Address: _____

Telephone: _____

Date: _____

Medical Consent Form

In case of emergency, _____ has my consent to authorize medical care for my child(ren) listed below:

_____   _____

_____   _____

_____   _____

Our family physician is: _____

His/Her address is: _____

His/Her telephone # is: _____

Our hospital preference is: _____

Allergies: _____

Contact me immediately at: _____

If unable to contact me, please call:

_____ @ _____
            Name   Telephone

_____ @ _____
            Name   Telephone

Signed by

Name: _____

Address: _____

Telephone: _____

Date: _____

Medical Consent Form

In case of emergency, _____ has my consent to authorize medical care for my child(ren) listed below:

_____   _____

_____   _____

_____   _____

Our family physician is: _____

His/Her address is: _____

His/Her telephone # is: _____

Our hospital preference is: _____

Allergies: _____

Contact me immediately at: _____

If unable to contact me, please call:

_____ @ _____
                Name   Telephone

_____ @ _____
                Name   Telephone

Signed by

Name: _____

Address: _____

Telephone: _____

Date: _____

Medical Consent Form

In case of emergency, _____ has my consent to authorize medical care for my child(ren) listed below:

_____   _____

_____   _____

_____   _____

Our family physician is: _____

His/Her address is: _____

His/Her telephone # is: _____

Our hospital preference is: _____

Allergies: _____

Contact me immediately at: _____

If unable to contact me, please call:

_____ @ _____
          Name   Telephone

_____ @ _____
          Name   Telephone

Signed by

Name: _____

Address: _____

Telephone: _____

Date: _____

Medical Consent Form

In case of emergency, _____ has my consent to authorize medical care for my child(ren) listed below:

_____   _____

_____   _____

_____   _____

Our family physician is: _____

His/Her address is: _____

His/Her telephone # is: _____

Our hospital preference is: _____

Allergies: _____

Contact me immediately at: _____

If unable to contact me, please call:

_____ @ _____
           Name   Telephone

_____ @ _____
           Name   Telephone

Signed by

Name: _____

Address: _____

Telephone: _____

Date: _____

Medical Consent Form

In case of emergency, _____ has my consent to authorize medical care for my child(ren) listed below:

_____   _____

_____   _____

_____   _____

Our family physician is: _____

His/Her address is: _____

His/Her telephone # is: _____

Our hospital preference is: _____

Allergies: _____

Contact me immediately at: _____

If unable to contact me, please call:

_____ @ _____
              Name   Telephone

_____ @ _____
              Name   Telephone

Signed by

Name: _____

Address: _____

Telephone: _____

Date: _____

Medical Consent Form

In case of emergency, _____ has my consent to authorize medical care for my child(ren) listed below:

_____   _____

_____   _____

_____   _____

Our family physician is: _____

His/Her address is: _____

His/Her telephone # is: _____

Our hospital preference is: _____

Allergies: _____

Contact me immediately at: _____

If unable to contact me, please call:

_____ @ _____
         Name   Telephone

_____ @ _____
         Name   Telephone

Signed by

Name: _____

Address: _____

Telephone: _____

Date: _____

Medical Consent Form

In case of emergency, _____ has my consent to authorize medical care for my child(ren) listed below:

_____   _____

_____   _____

_____   _____

Our family physician is: _____

His/Her address is: _____

His/Her telephone # is: _____

Our hospital preference is: _____

Allergies: _____

Contact me immediately at: _____

If unable to contact me, please call:

_____ @ _____
        Name   Telephone

_____ @ _____
        Name   Telephone

Signed by

Name: _____

Address: _____

Telephone: _____

Date: _____

Medical Consent Form

In case of emergency, _____ has my consent to authorize medical care for my child(ren) listed below:

_____   _____

_____   _____

_____   _____

Our family physician is: _____

His/Her address is: _____

His/Her telephone # is: _____

Our hospital preference is: _____

Allergies: _____

Contact me immediately at: _____

If unable to contact me, please call:

_____ @ _____
          Name   Telephone

_____ @ _____
          Name   Telephone

Signed by

Name: _____

Address: _____

Telephone: _____

Date: _____

Medical Consent Form

In case of emergency, _____ has my consent to authorize medical care for my child(ren) listed below:

_____   _____

_____   _____

_____   _____

Our family physician is: _____

His/Her address is: _____

His/Her telephone # is: _____

Our hospital preference is: _____

Allergies: _____

Contact me immediately at: _____

If unable to contact me, please call:

_____ @ _____
           Name   Telephone

_____ @ _____
           Name   Telephone

Signed by

Name: _____

Address: _____

Telephone: _____

Date: _____

Medical Consent Form

In case of emergency, _____ has my consent to authorize medical care for my child(ren) listed below:

_____   _____

_____   _____

_____   _____

Our family physician is: _____

His/Her address is: _____

His/Her telephone # is: _____

Our hospital preference is: _____

Allergies: _____

Contact me immediately at: _____

If unable to contact me, please call:

_____ @ _____
         Name   Telephone

_____ @ _____
         Name   Telephone

Signed by

Name: _____

Address: _____

Telephone: _____

Date: _____

Medical Consent Form

In case of emergency, _____ has my consent to authorize medical care for my child(ren) listed below:

_____   _____

_____   _____

_____   _____

Our family physician is: _____

His/Her address is: _____

His/Her telephone # is: _____

Our hospital preference is: _____

Allergies: _____

Contact me immediately at: _____

If unable to contact me, please call:

_____ @ _____
              Name   Telephone

_____ @ _____
              Name   Telephone

Signed by

Name: _____

Address: _____

Telephone: _____

Date: _____

Medical Consent Form

In case of emergency, _____ has my consent to authorize medical care for my child(ren) listed below:

_____   _____

_____   _____

_____   _____

Our family physician is: _____

His/Her address is: _____

His/Her telephone # is: _____

Our hospital preference is: _____

Allergies: _____

Contact me immediately at: _____

If unable to contact me, please call:

_____ @ _____
         Name   Telephone

_____ @ _____
         Name   Telephone

Signed by

Name: _____

Address: _____

Telephone: _____

Date: _____

Medical Consent Form

In case of emergency, _____ has my consent to authorize medical care for my child(ren) listed below:

_____   _____

_____   _____

_____   _____

Our family physician is: _____

His/Her address is: _____

His/Her telephone # is: _____

Our hospital preference is: _____

Allergies: _____

Contact me immediately at: _____

If unable to contact me, please call:

_____ @ _____
        Name   Telephone

_____ @ _____
        Name   Telephone

Signed by

Name: _____

Address: _____

Telephone: _____

Date: _____

Medical Consent Form

In case of emergency, _____ has my consent to authorize medical care for my child(ren) listed below:

_____   _____

_____   _____

_____   _____

Our family physician is: _____

His/Her address is: _____

His/Her telephone # is: _____

Our hospital preference is: _____

Allergies: _____

Contact me immediately at: _____

If unable to contact me, please call:

_____ @ _____
          Name   Telephone

_____ @ _____
          Name   Telephone

Signed by

Name: _____

Address: _____

Telephone: _____

Date: _____

Medical Consent Form

In case of emergency, _____ has my consent to authorize medical care for my child(ren) listed below:

_____   _____

_____   _____

_____   _____

Our family physician is: _____

His/Her address is: _____

His/Her telephone # is: _____

Our hospital preference is: _____

Allergies: _____

Contact me immediately at: _____

If unable to contact me, please call:

_____ @ _____
        Name   Telephone

_____ @ _____
        Name   Telephone

Signed by

Name: _____

Address: _____

Telephone: _____

Date: _____

Medical Consent Form

In case of emergency, _____ has my consent to authorize medical care for my child(ren) listed below:

_____   _____

_____   _____

_____   _____

Our family physician is: _____

His/Her address is: _____

His/Her telephone # is: _____

Our hospital preference is: _____

Allergies: _____

Contact me immediately at: _____

If unable to contact me, please call:

_____ @ _____
             Name   Telephone

_____ @ _____
             Name   Telephone

Signed by

Name: _____

Address: _____

Telephone: _____

Date: _____

Medical Consent Form

In case of emergency, _____ has my consent to authorize medical care for my child(ren) listed below:

_____   _____

_____   _____

_____   _____

Our family physician is: _____

His/Her address is: _____

His/Her telephone # is: _____

Our hospital preference is: _____

Allergies: _____

Contact me immediately at: _____

If unable to contact me, please call:

_____ @ _____
             Name   Telephone

_____ @ _____
             Name   Telephone

Signed by

Name: _____

Address: _____

Telephone: _____

Date: _____

Medical Consent Form

In case of emergency, _____ has my consent to authorize medical care for my child(ren) listed below:

_____   _____

_____   _____

_____   _____

Our family physician is: _____

His/Her address is: _____

His/Her telephone # is: _____

Our hospital preference is: _____

Allergies: _____

Contact me immediately at: _____

If unable to contact me, please call:

_____ @ _____
         Name   Telephone

_____ @ _____
         Name   Telephone

Signed by

Name: _____

Address: _____

Telephone: _____

Date: _____

Medical Consent Form

In case of emergency, _____ has my consent to authorize medical care for my child(ren) listed below:

_____   _____

_____   _____

_____   _____

Our family physician is: _____

His/Her address is: _____

His/Her telephone # is: _____

Our hospital preference is: _____

Allergies: _____

Contact me immediately at: _____

If unable to contact me, please call:

_____ @ _____
           Name   Telephone

_____ @ _____
           Name   Telephone

Signed by

Name: _____

Address: _____

Telephone: _____

Date: _____

Medical Consent Form

In case of emergency, _____ has my consent to authorize medical care for my child(ren) listed below:

_____   _____

_____   _____

_____   _____

Our family physician is: _____

His/Her address is: _____

His/Her telephone # is: _____

Our hospital preference is: _____

Allergies: _____

Contact me immediately at: _____

If unable to contact me, please call:

_____ @ _____
            Name   Telephone

_____ @ _____
            Name   Telephone

Signed by

Name: _____

Address: _____

Telephone: _____

Date: _____

Medical Consent Form

In case of emergency, _____ has my consent to authorize medical care for my child(ren) listed below:

_____   _____

_____   _____

_____   _____

Our family physician is: _____

His/Her address is: _____

His/Her telephone # is: _____

Our hospital preference is: _____

Allergies: _____

Contact me immediately at: _____

If unable to contact me, please call:

_____ @ _____
             Name   Telephone

_____ @ _____
             Name   Telephone

Signed by

Name: _____

Address: _____

Telephone: _____

Date: _____

Medical Consent Form

In case of emergency, _____ has my consent to authorize medical care for my child(ren) listed below:

_____   _____

_____   _____

_____   _____

Our family physician is: _____

His/Her address is: _____

His/Her telephone # is: _____

Our hospital preference is: _____

Allergies: _____

Contact me immediately at: _____

If unable to contact me, please call:

_____ @ _____
          Name   Telephone

_____ @ _____
          Name   Telephone

Signed by

Name: _____

Address: _____

Telephone: _____

Date: _____

Medical Consent Form

In case of emergency, _____ has my consent to authorize medical care for my child(ren) listed below:

_____   _____

_____   _____

_____   _____

Our family physician is: _____

His/Her address is: _____

His/Her telephone # is: _____

Our hospital preference is: _____

Allergies: _____

Contact me immediately at: _____

If unable to contact me, please call:

_____ @ _____
          Name   Telephone

_____ @ _____
          Name   Telephone

Signed by

Name: _____

Address: _____

Telephone: _____

Date: _____

Medical Consent Form

In case of emergency, _____ has my consent to authorize medical care for my child(ren) listed below:

_____ _____

_____ _____

_____ _____

Our family physician is: _____

His/Her address is: _____

His/Her telephone # is: _____

Our hospital preference is: _____

Allergies: _____

Contact me immediately at: _____

If unable to contact me, please call:

_____ @ _____
            Name   Telephone

_____ @ _____
            Name   Telephone

Signed by

Name: _____

Address: _____

Telephone: _____

Date: _____

Medical Consent Form

In case of emergency, _____ has my consent to authorize medical care for my child(ren) listed below:

_____   _____

_____   _____

_____   _____

Our family physician is: _____

His/Her address is: _____

His/Her telephone # is: _____

Our hospital preference is: _____

Allergies: _____

Contact me immediately at: _____

If unable to contact me, please call:

_____ @ _____
          Name   Telephone

_____ @ _____
          Name   Telephone

Signed by

Name: _____

Address: _____

Telephone: _____

Date: _____

Medical Consent Form

In case of emergency, _____ has my consent to authorize medical care for my child(ren) listed below:

_____   _____

_____   _____

_____   _____

Our family physician is: _____

His/Her address is: _____

His/Her telephone # is: _____

Our hospital preference is: _____

Allergies: _____

Contact me immediately at: _____

If unable to contact me, please call:

_____ @ _____
Name   Telephone

_____ @ _____
Name   Telephone

Signed by

Name: _____

Address: _____

Telephone: _____

Date: _____

Medical Consent Form

In case of emergency, _____ has my consent to authorize medical care for my child(ren) listed below:

_____   _____

_____   _____

_____   _____

Our family physician is: _____

His/Her address is: _____

His/Her telephone # is: _____

Our hospital preference is: _____

Allergies: _____

Contact me immediately at: _____

If unable to contact me, please call:

_____ @ _____
          Name   Telephone

_____ @ _____
          Name   Telephone

Signed by

Name: _____

Address: _____

Telephone: _____

Date: _____

Medical Consent Form

In case of emergency, _____ has my consent to authorize medical care for my child(ren) listed below:

_____   _____

_____   _____

_____   _____

Our family physician is: _____

His/Her address is: _____

His/Her telephone # is: _____

Our hospital preference is: _____

Allergies: _____

Contact me immediately at: _____

If unable to contact me, please call:

_____ @ _____
              Name   Telephone

_____ @ _____
              Name   Telephone

Signed by

Name: _____

Address: _____

Telephone: _____

Date: _____

Medical Consent Form

In case of emergency, _____ has my consent to authorize medical care for my child(ren) listed below:

_____   _____

_____   _____

_____   _____

Our family physician is: _____

His/Her address is: _____

His/Her telephone # is: _____

Our hospital preference is: _____

Allergies: _____

Contact me immediately at: _____

If unable to contact me, please call:

_____ @ _____
         Name   Telephone

_____ @ _____
         Name   Telephone

Signed by

Name: _____

Address: _____

Telephone: _____

Date: _____

Medical Consent Form

In case of emergency, _____ has my consent to authorize medical care for my child(ren) listed below:

_____   _____

_____   _____

_____   _____

Our family physician is: _____

His/Her address is: _____

His/Her telephone # is: _____

Our hospital preference is: _____

Allergies: _____

Contact me immediately at: _____

If unable to contact me, please call:

_____ @ _____
            Name   Telephone

_____ @ _____
            Name   Telephone

Signed by

Name: _____

Address: _____

Telephone: _____

Date: _____

Medical Consent Form

In case of emergency, _____ has my consent to authorize medical care for my child(ren) listed below:

_____   _____

_____   _____

_____   _____

Our family physician is: _____

His/Her address is: _____

His/Her telephone # is: _____

Our hospital preference is: _____

Allergies: _____

Contact me immediately at: _____

If unable to contact me, please call:

_____ @ _____
          Name   Telephone

_____ @ _____
          Name   Telephone

Signed by

Name: _____

Address: _____

Telephone: _____

Date: _____

Medical Consent Form

In case of emergency, _____ has my consent to authorize medical care for my child(ren) listed below:

_____   _____

_____   _____

_____   _____

Our family physician is: _____

His/Her address is: _____

His/Her telephone # is: _____

Our hospital preference is: _____

Allergies: _____

Contact me immediately at: _____

If unable to contact me, please call:

_____ @ _____
           Name   Telephone

_____ @ _____
           Name   Telephone

Signed by

Name: _____

Address: _____

Telephone: _____

Date: _____

Medical Consent Form

In case of emergency, _____ has my consent to authorize medical care for my child(ren) listed below:

_____   _____

_____   _____

_____   _____

Our family physician is: _____

His/Her address is: _____

His/Her telephone # is: _____

Our hospital preference is: _____

Allergies: _____

Contact me immediately at: _____

If unable to contact me, please call:

_____ @ _____
          Name   Telephone

_____ @ _____
          Name   Telephone

Signed by

Name: _____

Address: _____

Telephone: _____

Date: _____

Medical Consent Form

In case of emergency, _____ has my consent to authorize medical care for my child(ren) listed below:

_____   _____

_____   _____

_____   _____

Our family physician is: _____

His/Her address is: _____

His/Her telephone # is: _____

Our hospital preference is: _____

Allergies: _____

Contact me immediately at: _____

If unable to contact me, please call:

_____ @ _____
               Name   Telephone

_____ @ _____
               Name   Telephone

Signed by

Name: _____

Address: _____

Telephone: _____

Date: _____

Medical Consent Form

In case of emergency, _____ has my consent to authorize medical care for my child(ren) listed below:

_____ _____

_____ _____

_____ _____

Our family physician is: _____

His/Her address is: _____

His/Her telephone # is: _____

Our hospital preference is: _____

Allergies: _____

Contact me immediately at: _____

If unable to contact me, please call:

_____ @ _____
Name   Telephone

_____ @ _____
Name   Telephone

Signed by

Name: _____

Address: _____

Telephone: _____

Date: _____

Medical Consent Form

In case of emergency, _____ has my consent to authorize medical care for my child(ren) listed below:

_____   _____

_____   _____

_____   _____

Our family physician is: _____

His/Her address is: _____

His/Her telephone # is: _____

Our hospital preference is: _____

Allergies: _____

Contact me immediately at: _____

If unable to contact me, please call:

_____ @ _____
            Name   Telephone

_____ @ _____
            Name   Telephone

Signed by

Name: _____

Address: _____

Telephone: _____

Date: _____

Medical Consent Form

In case of emergency, _____ has my consent to authorize medical care for my child(ren) listed below:

_____   _____

_____   _____

_____   _____

Our family physician is: _____

His/Her address is: _____

His/Her telephone # is: _____

Our hospital preference is: _____

Allergies: _____

Contact me immediately at: _____

If unable to contact me, please call:

_____ @ _____
         Name   Telephone

_____ @ _____
         Name   Telephone

Signed by

Name: _____

Address: _____

Telephone: _____

Date: _____

Medical Consent Form

In case of emergency, _____ has my consent to authorize medical care for my child(ren) listed below:

_____   _____

_____   _____

_____   _____

Our family physician is: _____

His/Her address is: _____

His/Her telephone # is: _____

Our hospital preference is: _____

Allergies: _____

Contact me immediately at: _____

If unable to contact me, please call:

_____ @ _____
          Name   Telephone

_____ @ _____
          Name   Telephone

Signed by

Name: _____

Address: _____

Telephone: _____

Date: _____

Medical Consent Form

In case of emergency, _____ has my consent to authorize medical care for my child(ren) listed below:

_____   _____

_____   _____

_____   _____

Our family physician is: _____

His/Her address is: _____

His/Her telephone # is: _____

Our hospital preference is: _____

Allergies: _____

Contact me immediately at: _____

If unable to contact me, please call:

_____ @ _____
              Name   Telephone

_____ @ _____
              Name   Telephone

Signed by

Name: _____

Address: _____

Telephone: _____

Date: _____

Medical Consent Form

In case of emergency, _____ has my consent to authorize medical care for my child(ren) listed below:

_____   _____

_____   _____

_____   _____

Our family physician is: _____

His/Her address is: _____

His/Her telephone # is: _____

Our hospital preference is: _____

Allergies: _____

Contact me immediately at: _____

If unable to contact me, please call:

_____ @ _____
            Name   Telephone

_____ @ _____
            Name   Telephone

Signed by

Name: _____

Address: _____

Telephone: _____

Date: _____

Medical Consent Form

In case of emergency, _____ has my consent to authorize medical care for my child(ren) listed below:

_____   _____

_____   _____

_____   _____

Our family physician is: _____

His/Her address is: _____

His/Her telephone # is: _____

Our hospital preference is: _____

Allergies: _____

Contact me immediately at: _____

If unable to contact me, please call:

_____ @ _____
          Name   Telephone

_____ @ _____
          Name   Telephone

Signed by

Name: _____

Address: _____

Telephone: _____

Date: _____

Medical Consent Form

In case of emergency, _____ has my consent to authorize medical care for my child(ren) listed below:

_____   _____

_____   _____

_____   _____

Our family physician is: _____

His/Her address is: _____

His/Her telephone # is: _____

Our hospital preference is: _____

Allergies: _____

Contact me immediately at: _____

If unable to contact me, please call:

_____ @ _____
         Name   Telephone

_____ @ _____
         Name   Telephone

Signed by

Name: _____

Address: _____

Telephone: _____

Date: _____

Medical Consent Form

In case of emergency, _____ has my consent to authorize medical care for my child(ren) listed below:

_____   _____

_____   _____

_____   _____

Our family physician is: _____

His/Her address is: _____

His/Her telephone # is: _____

Our hospital preference is: _____

Allergies: _____

Contact me immediately at: _____

If unable to contact me, please call:

_____ @ _____
            Name   Telephone

_____ @ _____
            Name   Telephone

Signed by

Name: _____

Address: _____

Telephone: _____

Date: _____

Medical Consent Form

In case of emergency, _____ has my consent to authorize medical care for my child(ren) listed below:

_____   _____

_____   _____

_____   _____

Our family physician is: _____

His/Her address is: _____

His/Her telephone # is: _____

Our hospital preference is: _____

Allergies: _____

Contact me immediately at: _____

If unable to contact me, please call:

_____ @ _____
        Name   Telephone

_____ @ _____
        Name   Telephone

Signed by

Name: _____

Address: _____

Telephone: _____

Date: _____

Medical Consent Form

In case of emergency, _____ has my consent to authorize medical care for my child(ren) listed below:

_____   _____

_____   _____

_____   _____

Our family physician is: _____

His/Her address is: _____

His/Her telephone # is: _____

Our hospital preference is: _____

Allergies: _____

Contact me immediately at: _____

If unable to contact me, please call:

_____ @ _____
             Name   Telephone

_____ @ _____
             Name   Telephone

Signed by

Name: _____

Address: _____

Telephone: _____

Date: _____

Medical Consent Form

In case of emergency, _____ has my consent to authorize medical care for my child(ren) listed below:

_____   _____

_____   _____

_____   _____

Our family physician is: _____

His/Her address is: _____

His/Her telephone # is: _____

Our hospital preference is: _____

Allergies: _____

Contact me immediately at: _____

If unable to contact me, please call:

_____ @ _____
      Name   Telephone

_____ @ _____
      Name   Telephone

Signed by

Name: _____

Address: _____

Telephone: _____

Date: _____

Medical Consent Form

In case of emergency, _____ has my consent to authorize medical care for my child(ren) listed below:

_____   _____

_____   _____

_____   _____

Our family physician is: _____

His/Her address is: _____

His/Her telephone # is: _____

Our hospital preference is: _____

Allergies: _____

Contact me immediately at: _____

If unable to contact me, please call:

_____ @ _____
             Name   Telephone

_____ @ _____
             Name   Telephone

Signed by

Name: _____

Address: _____

Telephone: _____

Date: _____

Medical Consent Form

In case of emergency, _____ has my consent to authorize medical care for my child(ren) listed below:

_____   _____

_____   _____

_____   _____

Our family physician is: _____

His/Her address is: _____

His/Her telephone # is: _____

Our hospital preference is: _____

Allergies: _____

Contact me immediately at: _____

If unable to contact me, please call:

_____ @ _____
         Name   Telephone

_____ @ _____
         Name   Telephone

Signed by

Name: _____

Address: _____

Telephone: _____

Date: _____

Medical Consent Form

In case of emergency, _____ has my consent to authorize medical care for my child(ren) listed below:

_____   _____

_____   _____

_____   _____

Our family physician is: _____

His/Her address is: _____

His/Her telephone # is: _____

Our hospital preference is: _____

Allergies: _____

Contact me immediately at: _____

If unable to contact me, please call:

_____ @ _____
          Name   Telephone

_____ @ _____
          Name   Telephone

Signed by

Name: _____

Address: _____

Telephone: _____

Date: _____

Medical Consent Form

In case of emergency, _____ has my consent to authorize medical care for my child(ren) listed below:

_____   _____

_____   _____

_____   _____

Our family physician is: _____

His/Her address is: _____

His/Her telephone # is: _____

Our hospital preference is: _____

Allergies: _____

Contact me immediately at: _____

If unable to contact me, please call:

_____ @ _____
         Name   Telephone

_____ @ _____
         Name   Telephone

Signed by

Name: _____

Address: _____

Telephone: _____

Date: _____

Medical Consent Form

In case of emergency, _____ has my consent to authorize medical care for my child(ren) listed below:

_____   _____

_____   _____

_____   _____

Our family physician is: _____

His/Her address is: _____

His/Her telephone # is: _____

Our hospital preference is: _____

Allergies: _____

Contact me immediately at: _____

If unable to contact me, please call:

_____ @ _____
        Name   Telephone

_____ @ _____
        Name   Telephone

Signed by

Name: _____

Address: _____

Telephone: _____

Date: _____

Medical Consent Form

In case of emergency, _____ has my consent to authorize medical care for my child(ren) listed below:

_____   _____

_____   _____

_____   _____

Our family physician is: _____

His/Her address is: _____

His/Her telephone # is: _____

Our hospital preference is: _____

Allergies: _____

Contact me immediately at: _____

If unable to contact me, please call:

_____ @ _____
        Name   Telephone

_____ @ _____
        Name   Telephone

Signed by

Name: _____

Address: _____

Telephone: _____

Date: _____

Medical Consent Form

In case of emergency, _____ has my consent to authorize medical care for my child(ren) listed below:

_____   _____

_____   _____

_____   _____

Our family physician is: _____

His/Her address is: _____

His/Her telephone # is: _____

Our hospital preference is: _____

Allergies: _____

Contact me immediately at: _____

If unable to contact me, please call:

_____ @ _____
            Name   Telephone

_____ @ _____
            Name   Telephone

Signed by

Name: _____

Address: _____

Telephone: _____

Date: _____

Medical Consent Form

In case of emergency, _____ has my consent to authorize medical care for my child(ren) listed below:

_____   _____

_____   _____

_____   _____

Our family physician is: _____

His/Her address is: _____

His/Her telephone # is: _____

Our hospital preference is: _____

Allergies: _____

Contact me immediately at: _____

If unable to contact me, please call:

_____ @ _____
         Name   Telephone

_____ @ _____
         Name   Telephone

Signed by

Name: _____

Address: _____

Telephone: _____

Date: _____

Medical Consent Form

In case of emergency, _____ has my consent to authorize medical care for my child(ren) listed below:

_____   _____

_____   _____

_____   _____

Our family physician is: _____

His/Her address is: _____

His/Her telephone # is: _____

Our hospital preference is: _____

Allergies: _____

Contact me immediately at: _____

If unable to contact me, please call:

_____ @ _____
            Name   Telephone

_____ @ _____
            Name   Telephone

Signed by

Name: _____

Address: _____

Telephone: _____

Date: _____

Medical Consent Form

In case of emergency, _____ has my consent to authorize medical care for my child(ren) listed below:

_____   _____

_____   _____

_____   _____

Our family physician is: _____

His/Her address is: _____

His/Her telephone # is: _____

Our hospital preference is: _____

Allergies: _____

Contact me immediately at: _____

If unable to contact me, please call:

_____ @ _____
        Name   Telephone

_____ @ _____
        Name   Telephone

Signed by

Name: _____

Address: _____

Telephone: _____

Date: _____

Medical Consent Form

In case of emergency, _____ has my consent to authorize medical care for my child(ren) listed below:

_____   _____

_____   _____

_____   _____

Our family physician is: _____

His/Her address is: _____

His/Her telephone # is: _____

Our hospital preference is: _____

Allergies: _____

Contact me immediately at: _____

If unable to contact me, please call:

_____ @ _____
              Name   Telephone

_____ @ _____
              Name   Telephone

Signed by

Name: _____

Address: _____

Telephone: _____

Date: _____

Medical Consent Form

In case of emergency, _____ has my consent to authorize medical care for my child(ren) listed below:

_____   _____

_____   _____

_____   _____

Our family physician is: _____

His/Her address is: _____

His/Her telephone # is: _____

Our hospital preference is: _____

Allergies: _____

Contact me immediately at: _____

If unable to contact me, please call:

_____ @ _____
          Name   Telephone

_____ @ _____
          Name   Telephone

Signed by

Name: _____

Address: _____

Telephone: _____

Date: _____

Medical Consent Form

In case of emergency, _____ has my consent to authorize medical care for my child(ren) listed below:

_____   _____

_____   _____

_____   _____

Our family physician is: _____

His/Her address is: _____

His/Her telephone # is: _____

Our hospital preference is: _____

Allergies: _____

Contact me immediately at: _____

If unable to contact me, please call:

_____ @ _____
            Name   Telephone

_____ @ _____
            Name   Telephone

Signed by

Name: _____

Address: _____

Telephone: _____

Date: _____

Medical Consent Form

In case of emergency, _____ has my consent to authorize medical care for my child(ren) listed below:

_____   _____

_____   _____

_____   _____

Our family physician is: _____

His/Her address is: _____

His/Her telephone # is: _____

Our hospital preference is: _____

Allergies: _____

Contact me immediately at: _____

If unable to contact me, please call:

_____ @ _____
        Name   Telephone

_____ @ _____
        Name   Telephone

Signed by

Name: _____

Address: _____

Telephone: _____

Date: _____

Medical Consent Form

In case of emergency, _____ has my consent to authorize medical care for my child(ren) listed below:

_____   _____

_____   _____

_____   _____

Our family physician is: _____

His/Her address is: _____

His/Her telephone # is: _____

Our hospital preference is: _____

Allergies: _____

Contact me immediately at: _____

If unable to contact me, please call:

_____ @ _____
              Name   Telephone

_____ @ _____
              Name   Telephone

Signed by

Name: _____

Address: _____

Telephone: _____

Date: _____

www.ingramcontent.com/pod-product-compliance
Lightning Source LLC
Chambersburg PA
CBHW081118180526
45170CB00008B/2902